MEN On PAUSE

A MAN'S GUIDE TO UNDERSTANDING MENOPAUSE

BY LELITIA LANE

Copyright © 2017 Lelitia Lane. All rights reserved.

ISBN-13: 978-1976347245
ISBN-10: 1976347246

The information in this book is not intended or implied to be a substitute for professional medical advice, diagnosis or treatment. Consult your physician before starting any supplements or dietary changes.

Table of Contents

ACKNOWLEDGMENTS III

MENOPAUSE: WHAT IS IT, REALLY??? V

GET READY FOR THE RIDE! 1

PERSONAL SUMMERS 5

SEX-ON-PAUSE 13

CRAZY LADY!?! 21

WEIGHT ON!! 27

HANG IN THERE!! 31

ABOUT THE AUTHOR 35

REFERENCES 36

Acknowledgments

I would like to thank my AWESOME husband, Roland Lane Jr., for putting up with me and not leaving me during this new phase in our lives, called menopause.

I also thank our children, Rolanda, Morgan, Jene', Jeffery, Jaden, and Jalen, because they have to feel the wrath of menopause.

To my beautiful mother, Doris Champion Johnson, words cannot express how thankful and grateful I am for you being my mom. You taught me so many things. Thanks for teaching me that there is nothing I "CAN'T DO." I am sorry you couldn't be here to see me finish this book.

I also thank my mother- and father-in-law, Rachel and Roland Lane Sr., for raising a phenomenal son who is par excellence.

I thank my sister Trecye, her husband Kevin, and her children Doriann and Darius, for always encouraging and supporting me forever.

I thank my brother Thaddeus, his wife Tina, and my nephews Thaddeus and Tristen, for loving and supporting me.

A special thanks and shout out to Daveda Platt. You "rock!" Thanks for your encouragement and support. You walked me through this process with grace and professionalism. I am truly grateful.

I love you all!!!

Most of all, I would like to thank my Lord and Savior Jesus Christ for not giving up on me. It took me some time to realize and understand HIS plan and purpose for my life. To God be the Glory!!!

Introduction
MENOPAUSE: WHAT IS IT, REALLY???

Menopause is a natural part of every woman's life. It's a normal and innate experience that usually occurs in women between the ages of 45 to 55, with an average age of 51. Simply put, menopause is the time in a woman's life when her period or menstrual cycle ends. Menopause is complete when 12 consecutive months have gone by without a menstrual period. The body goes through changes that no longer allow a woman to get pregnant.

At menopause, the ovaries stop producing the female hormones, estrogen and progesterone. This can cause UNDESIRABLE symptoms and can also affect a woman's health. Symptoms can occur four to five years before menopause begins and remain several years after. Menopause is a turning point—not a disease—and it can have a big impact on a woman's well-being.

This book was written to inform and encourage men all over the world who have women in their lives who are experiencing this beast, called menopause. I pray this book will bring you great insight and give you a better understanding of what's going on in your wife or your girlfriend's life. In this book, I share some things that my husband and I went through and, at this time, are still going through with perimenopause, the onset and symptoms of menopause, and menopause itself.

Chapter One
GET READY FOR THE RIDE!

My husband often says, "If mama's not happy, ain't nobody happy!" This thing called menopause will upset your whole household. There's something going on inside of mama like a hurricane, that mama doesn't understand. And everything and everybody that gets in her path has to suffer her wrath. After the storm, you've become collateral damage without her even knowing it.

Menopause may be a natural part of a woman's life, but its cause and effects happen to affect not only her life, but also her husband and her loved ones as well. It seems menopause affects husbands or men more than women. Isn't it funny how the words MENopause and MENstruation both have the prefix "MEN," and that's who suffers from the effects of this monumental change in life the most (besides the woman, of course).

Men, you thought PMS was bad—menopause will add another notch to your survivor belt! I don't know why women have to go through the things that we do. I guess it's part of the punishment from Eve eating the forbidden fruit. LOL!! Menopause is a natural part of aging, and every woman's experience with it is different. You've got to know that this is not your woman having a tantrum, pity party or just going *slap off*. It's a serious thing going on within her, and she really has no clue what's happening or how to explain it.

I remember feeling different and knowing that something was going on with me. I would burst out crying at times, and then I would go off on anyone who came in my path. Most of the time, that person would be my husband. Poor thing. He was so confused. Sometimes the things I would do and say would hurt him, and he would just shut down. He'd often say, "What happened to you? You were so sweet when I married you, and that was one of the reasons why I married you!" I would feel so bad after showing out and him quoting that infamous line. But what was happening was the onset of menopause. My children were not spared either. I remember so well one day, after going off about something simple, my daughter Morgan said, "Mama what's wrong with you??? You are going off on us for nothing. Are you OK?" After coming to myself, I felt so ashamed and small. I started thinking to myself; *what's really going on?*

> "Some of the symptoms of menopause include, mood swings, depression, anxiety, irritability, fatigue, crying spells, loss of memory, blowing up like a hand grenade (in my own words); as well as hot flashes, night sweats, weight gain, and no sexual desire..."

Some of the symptoms of menopause include, mood swings, depression, anxiety, irritability, fatigue, crying spells, loss of memory, blowing up like a hand grenade (in my own words); as well as hot flashes, night sweats, weight gain, and no sexual desire, which we will discuss later in this book. It seemed like I was experiencing ALL of these symptoms at once!

At the time, I knew something was wrong, but I didn't understand what was going on. I asked both my primary care doctor and my gynecologist if I was going through menopause, and they both said no and that I was too young to be going through menopause. Both of my doctors happen to be around the same age as I am, so I guess these things were not happening to them. I was about 44 or 45 when the craziness began. Several years went by and I continued asking, but the answer was still the same. Finally, when I was about 47, after much asking and complaining from my husband and me, my gynecologist drew some blood and ran some tests. And guess what she found out!!!??? I was perimenopausal. Well, I had been saying it for over three years, but nobody believed me! After my doctor gave us the results, I immediately had her explain to my husband that all the craziness was not me, but the menopause. I think he was ready to send me away to the nearest mental institution…you know… the place where they put people in padded rooms with straitjackets on them!?

Menopause is an emotional roller coaster ride. During the month, one moment you're up, the next moment you're down, sometimes you're OK and then there are times when you're an emotional wreck. Even though there's no menstrual cycle, your body and hormones still carry on as if you are having one, as far as your emotions are concerned. There are two things that most women have in common, and that is dreading having to deal monthly with our periods, and that we all can't wait until it goes away for good. We just don't realize that the process of it going away is just as agonizing as it is to keep it.

In today's society, women are bragging about how they are aging and not looking like their age. You know the saying, "50 is the new 40" and "40 is the new 30?" Although we are healthier, working out, eating right, looking fabulous and, in some cases, living longer, there is one thing we can't change or manage with exercise or healthy eating—menopause. Our bodies are screaming, "I'm going through the change!" and it's taking over whether we're ready for it or not.

Chapter Two
PERSONAL SUMMERS

"Keep a livin," are the words that use to come out of my aunt's mouth when I would question her about putting her head in the freezer every 15 minutes. She would break out in a great sweat, and I didn't know what was going on. My other aunt would break out too, and I thought it was the heat because they would be in the kitchen helping my mom cook every Sunday after church. Well, it wasn't the heat in the kitchen, but they were definitely on FIRE!!! A personal fire. One that I didn't want to have anything to do with. I even prayed that it wouldn't come upon me.

"Hot flash" is the politically correct term for that type of fire. Hot flash is one of the most common symptoms and the most hated of menopause. This symptom really drives a woman crazy. It's so frustrating. An article on DoctorOz.com describes it, saying:

> "Hot flashes typically begin as a sudden sensation of heat on the face and upper chest, and spreads over the body. It can be pretty intense, lasting between two and four minutes, followed by profuse sweating. As if that weren't enough, many women also have chills and shivering. Physiologically, a hot flash happens for the same reason that you sweat in a sauna… the body is trying to cool down. The difference is, you don't really need to cool down, but your menopausal brain thinks you do."

The article continues, "The human body is meant to be roughly 98.6 degrees. It has functions in place to help regulate our temperature. If you go outside in the winter without your coat, you're going to shiver to generate heat. You sweat when you exercise to cool your body down. The part of the brain that keeps your body at the right temperature is known as the thermoregulatory zone. But during menopause, the thermoregulatory zone gets too sensitive, resulting in a hot flash even when the body doesn't really need to cool down."

My children often joke that my body temperature is bi-polar, because one minute I'm burning up, then the next minute I'm freezing. Although the hot flash lasts a few minutes, it feels like forever. Imagine your body temperature is steaming hot, like a pot of boiling water, then the next second, your body feels like you've been thrown into a freezer 10 degrees below zero, and all of this happening in a matter of minutes. Sometimes it's really overwhelming. I can be dressed and ready to go, and before I get to where I'm going, I want to take a bath again.

I know my husband hates to drive my car with me in it. He never says it, but I believe he does. I say this because, the button on the passenger side that opens and closes the window is broken and while he's driving, he has to let down the window because I'm hot—and seconds later, I ask him to let it back up because I'm cold. In the winter, while the window is down, it takes away all of the heat, and everyone in the car freezes.

One winter here in Georgia, we had temperatures in the teens, and I was hanging out of the window sweating. This is an example of a car ride with us, and the process that goes on for the whole ride: "Let down the window, I'm hot. Thanks... Now, let up the window, I'm cold!!" *Crazy, right?* The same thing happens in the summer with the air conditioner. The summer I first started having flashes, I had the ceiling fan and the air conditioner on. My husband was so cold, he went to bed wearing a sweat suit and a skullcap! I really hate that my family has to suffer through this process, but I'm grateful that they support and put up with me.

There's a commercial that shows different women having hot flashes and taking off their clothes and jackets in their boardroom meetings and everyday life situations. Every time I see it, I just laugh because it's so true. One moment you have your clothes on and the next you're stripping them off.

Hot flashes are also terrible at night. One minute you want the covers on you, the next minute you're kicking them off. Sometimes it seems like, as soon as my husband wants to cuddle, I break out in a hot sweat and we have to go to our separate corners. There are nights when I wake up and my pajamas are drenched in sweat, then shortly after, I'm shaking because I am freezing. It's a miserable feeling and it can be so frustrating!!

Hot flashes can take a toll on your body. I recently started having heart palpitations at night. I thought I was going to have a heart attack. I would have a hot flash, and along with it, my heart would start beating really fast and I'd feel very jittery. I went to my doctor and told her that I was having two types of flashes; the regular ones, where I am hot and cold, and the other one, where my heart is beating very fast and I'd feel jittery along

> "There are nights when I wake up and my pajamas are drenched in sweat, then shortly after, I'm shaking because I am freezing. It's a miserable feeling and it can be so frustrating!!"

with being hot and cold. She told me that heart palpitations are very common in women who are having hot flashes.

The exact cause of flashes is still not entirely understood. This is hardly a new problem, and you would think that by now, someone would have come up with something better than a portable fan to fix it. However, there are some things that can be done to help minimize or curb the flashes. Some remedies won't take the flashes away totally, but it will calm them down and slow down the occurrences. For example, I love taking very hot showers, but when I get out of the shower, I immediately have a hot flash and I have to step back in the shower because I'm all sweaty. I learned the key to taking a great hot shower is to turn the water to cold before getting out of the shower. This takes the body temperature back down.

Some other things that can help curb hot flashes is what your girl eats. Tell her to STAY AWAY from CAFFEINE and SUGAR!!! These two ingredients will set off epic hot flashes, like lighting a barrel of fireworks for the grand finale at a 4th of July show! These two are not a girl's friend—they are definitely the enemy. Spicy foods and alcohol are things to avoid as well. There are some medicines out there that a doctor can prescribe, but sticking to natural remedies is much better. I got a prescription for my hot flashes, but it made all of my symptoms worse, and I thought I was going to lose my mind.

> "Tell her to STAY AWAY from CAFFEINE and SUGAR!!! These two ingredients will set off epic hot flashes, like lighting a barrel of fireworks for the grand finale at a 4th of July show!"

Black cohosh is one of the most widely used natural or alternative therapies for treatment of hot flashes. According to an article written in the INH Health Watch Newsletter, a new study shows that the herb fennel is safe and effective against menopause symptoms.

Here's a list of a few natural foods, vitamins or products that can help your lady win the battle of the flashes. They can be found at any store that carries natural foods and products.

SUPPLEMENTS	WHAT TO EAT	WHAT TO DRINK
Black Cohosh	Fruits	Water
Vitamin E & D	Dark Leafy Vegetables	Non-Dairy Beverages
Calcium	Whole Grains	Sage Tea
Fennel Seeds	Eggs	Green Tea
Flax Seeds	Soy	Green Juices or Smoothies

This information is not intended to be a substitute for professional medical advice, diagnosis or treatment. Always seek the advice of your physician before trying any supplements or dietary changes.

I haven't tried all of these foods or products, but they were highly recommended by people who have, and they say that these work. I decided to start a clean eating lifestyle, and I've noticed that I don't really have that many hot flashes anymore. If you're not sure how to begin clean eating, the Internet is a place where you can find many recipes and meal plans. Two of my favorite websites that can help you jump-start a clean eating lifestyle is emeal.com and pinterest.com.

There are many other things your woman can try, like exercise, acupuncture and yoga. Multiple studies have shown that women who exercise regularly have fewer hot flashes due to exercise-induced endorphin production. Losing extra weight (though menopause may cause women to gain weight and make it hard to lose) and eliminating cigarettes also makes a huge difference. Be aware that, the average woman can expect to experience moderate to severe hot flashes for about five years. About 20 percent will continue to have flashes for even longer (perhaps forever).

Please pray for the woman in your life. I once read an article that said men can have hot flashes too, so tread lightly and be supportive. Hot flashes are no fun, so when the woman in your life is sweating profusely, and it's not from working out, have mercy, and ask her if you can bring her a cold glass of water. I keep a cup filled with ice and water on the nightstand on my side of the bed, so when I start having a hot flash, the ice-cold glass of water helps put out the flames.

Patience is Key

Remember, hot flashes can be overwhelming, exhausting and cause great frustration. So much is going on in your lady's mind and in her body. It is important that you remain patient with her and make allowances for her shortcomings. The Word of God reminds us...

"Always be humble and gentle. Be patient with each other, making allowance for each other's faults because of your love." Ephesians 4:2 (New Living Translation)

Chapter Three
SEX-ON-PAUSE

Sex-On-Pause is what happens during menopause when the sexual part of your relationship is put on pause. The lack of sex can cause major damage to your relationship. There are three main things that can destroy a marriage, and they are; lack of communication, lack of money, and lack of sex. Menopause can wreak havoc on your marriage due to lack of sex and cause intimacy in your relationship to suffer more than anything else.

During this stage in life, for some women, sex is not a problem. As a matter of fact, their sex life gets turned up a notch. I heard in the past that, once a woman reached middle age, her sex life is better than it was when she was younger. I was oh so looking to be off the chain!! You know...having sex all the time, anywhere, swinging from the chandelier, trying different things and sneaking in spontaneous episodes... Well, unfortunately for me and thousands of other women, instead of "turning up" we "turned down." Sex becomes a big problem with menopause, because things are changing in our bodies.

There are two reasons why women shun sex during menopause— lack of sexual desire and painful sex. The lack of sexual desire has absolutely nothing to do with you personally and nothing to do with your wife not being attracted to you, or her not wanting to be with you sexually. You are still sexy, attractive and desirable, but her hormones are out of whack! You are still the man that she wants to be with and make love to, but there are times when the desire is just gone. *Where?* That's the question I want to know the answer to as well. If you find out where it is, let me know! According to Fitness Magazine, "decreased interest in sexual activity is often a sign of hormonal imbalance, which can cause both physical and emotional symptoms that have an effect on your sex life." This is the time to really call on God for help, because this process requires mercy and patience.

> *"This is the time to really call on God for help, because this process requires mercy and patience. Lack of sex can become a problem and put a strain on a marriage."*

Lack of sex can become a problem and put a strain on a marriage. *Can I just be honest and share something with you?* Not being able to perform sexually begins to mess with your wife and her womanhood. Let's be real for a minute. If a man is not able to perform sexually, it messes with his manhood. Some men have problems with sex too, because their bodies are not operating like it used to. Some men require the help of a little blue pill. So come on guys! Please give your girl a break and apply a little grace and mercy when she says, "not tonight."

If your woman is already struggling with who she is and self-esteem is something she's already dealing with, it takes the problem to a whole other level, adding self-doubt, depression and fear. She becomes afraid that her husband is going to leave because she's not "putting out" when he wants it. Once fear is in play, not trusting becomes an issue. *"Is he cheating?" "Will he leave me?"* All of this becomes a big issue in your marriage. Every woman wants to please her husband sexually and is willing to do whatever it takes to satisfy him.

When I started going through this process, I was unable to explain to my husband what was going on, I just knew there were a lot of nights he went to bed very unhappy!

Communication is key during this process, even when there's no clue to what's going on. It's sad, but true, some men cheat and leave during this time, so it's important to talk to your wife. There is a new trend now. Men are usually the ones who leave during this time, but according to healthywomen.org, a recent survey conducted by AARP Magazine showed that, "Over 60 percent of divorces were initiated by women in their 40s, 50s, and 60s—the menopause years." The culprit behind the divorces was lack of communication. So, start talking!! Encouragement and support is very important, because this is such a big change and process.

The second reason why women shun sex is because, during menopause, sex can be very painful. According to Fitness Magazine, "Approximately 50 percent of post-menopausal women experience vaginal dryness, which can make sex painful." If intercourse hurt you, you'd have a drop in your sexual desire, too! Once menopause sets in, the vagina becomes very dry and it's hard for a woman to get excited and lubricated in that area. The things you use to do—the foreplay, the touches and kisses—no longer gets the vagina stimulated. Now, it will take some extra work and communication to figure out how to make it possible for the vagina to produce the moisture needed to make it pleasurable for you and her.

> "The culprit behind the divorces was lack of communication. So, start talking!! Encouragement and support is very important, because this is such a big change and process."

Let me explain how painful the sex is. I asked God to give

me an example to give you a clear understanding of how it may feel to your wife. Have you ever had a rug burn? Or while playing baseball, slid into home plate and got a burn called a "cherry?" If the answer is yes, imagine getting a rug burn or a cherry on your penis! *Ouch!!!* It's like rubbing two dry sticks together—all you get is friction, burning, and tearing. Well, that's what happens to your wife during sex. In my case, most of the time I really didn't want to go through the pain, but out of fear of my husband going elsewhere, I went ahead and took the pain. You may not be thinking about leaving your wife, but the fear for her is still there, and it's real. The pain lasts for days, and if you have sex more than once in a night or days after, it's absolutely awful! The vagina needs time to heal. If you continue to have sex, it makes it worse, so it's easier to say, "no, not tonight...I'm tired," than to endure any more pain. Communication, again, is key. Your wife needs to explain her pain and the two of you need to figure out how to have sex that is still pleasurable to you both.

> *"You may not be thinking about leaving your wife, but the fear for her is still there, and it's real."*

There are products that can help with lubrication, like KY Jelly. You can also find healthy products on www.amazing-solutions.com, www.AloeCadabra.com and www.bermansexualhealth.com, to name a few. There are also some creative things you can do to help her get the moisture needed to make sex easy and pleasurable again.

Work out a plan. For example, when a couple is trying to get pregnant, the wife has to monitor or calculate when she is ovulating. Once she realizes she's ovulating, she goes to her husband and says, "It's time!! Let's get it on!" Your wife has to figure out when her body desires sex, then she can come to you and say, "It's time!! Let's get it on!"

Now, there may be times when you're not ready. At this point, get creative!! Pray and ask God to put the desire in both of you at the same time, and He will do it. I am a witness that He will. Take time out for intimacy. WebMD provides these great pointers:

> *"You can still show love and affection without having sex. Intimacy goes beyond sexual intercourse—it's not just sex. Intimacy is about closeness, about being together and about creating and maintaining a relationship. It's an important part of any relationship, with or without sexual intercourse. Enjoy your time together. Take walks, eat dinner by candlelight, or give each other back rubs. You might not be having intercourse, but you can still enjoy orgasms by exploring other forms of stimulation or by having outercourse. Outercourse is any form of sensual and sexual activity that does not involve the exchange of body fluids."*

Go ahead—try something new and different! Anything to keep your relationship new and fresh.

There are a lot of products for men to take to help with their libido, but not women. There are many studies being conducted and there are pills that women can take, but I wouldn't suggest meds. I suggest women do it naturally, through their diet.

There are other options to consider, such as counseling. Your doctor may refer you and your lady to a health professional who specializes in sexual dysfunction. The therapist may advise sexual counseling on an individual basis, with your partner or in a support group. This type of counseling can be very successful, even when it's done on a short-term basis.

My husband and I decided on a lifestyle change. We started

a clean eating lifestyle. This wasn't a diet or a fad; we simply changed what we ate. Little did we know, eating better would increase my sexual desire. Here I was, thinking that life was over, and just a change in what I was eating caused a great big change in my sex life. The Internet has tons of information about clean eating and there are some awesome recipes as well. Give it a try.

Here's a list of foods that can help a woman's libido:

Black Raspberries	Broccoli	Eggs
Cloves	Watermelon	Saffron
Figs	Ginseng	Iceberg Lettuce
Ginger	Dark Chocolate	Dark Leafy Greens

This information is not intended to be a substitute for professional medical advice, diagnosis or treatment. Always seek the advice of your physician before trying any supplements or dietary changes.

Good luck with figuring out the best way to maintain a healthy and great sex life for you and your lady!

A Prayer for Renewed Intimacy

(Pray this prayer. Insert your significant other's name in the blank.)

Father,

I pray that the sexual bond and intimacy between _____ and me will not be hindered or put on pause due to menopause. Help us not to give up on having intercourse. Give us a strategy that will make sex a joy and not a pain. Grant an everlasting open door of communication between us, so that we can be open and honest about our feelings and desires. I pray that we will find creative ways to enjoy each other intimately. I declare that our sexual encounters will be exhilarating and fulfilling! Thank you in advance for bringing us closer together. In Jesus' awesome name. Amen!!

Chapter Four
CRAZY LADY!?!

Your lady is NOT crazy!! I repeat—your lady is NOT crazy!!! One spring day about mid-morning, I'm staring at my face in the mirror, my hair is standing on top of my head, and I am looking quite crazy. I didn't know what was going on with me. I couldn't explain it, but I knew something wasn't right, so I called my doctor. I told her about the symptoms I was having and she gave me some medicine that was supposed to balance my hormones. Instead, it took my hormones to another level. I was already on an emotional rollercoaster, but the meds took me on the ride of my life. If it weren't for a close family friend praying for me that day I think my new home would have been at a mental institution.

Menopause comes with a lot of hormonal imbalances. Along with the normal cares and stress of living, menopause adds more wood to this fiery inferno called, "the issues of life." There are some times when I really feel like I'm going to lose my mind. I started wondering, "What's *really* going on?" I often feel like I'm about to have a nervous breakdown. It's really hard to explain actually what I feel. It's really weird. These feelings are ones that I pretty much keep to myself, because no one wants to think that they're crazy. And there are times when I really feel like I'm about to lose it! Once I realized that it was one of the many symptoms of menopause, a great sigh of relief came over me.

> WebMD.com describes, "Emotional changes are a normal part of menopause. There are a lot of women who feel down, blue, sad, irritable, anxious, moody, and some feel like a raving maniac. Many women experience unnerving changes in their emotions, memory and concentration during perimenopause and menopause, due to sudden shifts in hormones. Changes in estrogen and progesterone levels may cause mood swings. Drops in progesterone may cause increased irritability and moodiness. Menopause is a developmental milestone in a woman's life. It's sometimes referred to as adolescence in reverse. It's just like the onset of a woman's menstrual cycle."

The woman in your life may be experiencing some of this "craziness." It's a little scary because you don't know if you need to get professional help or if it will just pass. On top of everything else that's going on in our lives, from the start of the day until the end, we have to juggle and deal with taking care of our man's needs, the children's needs, household needs, and work, etc. Our needs are somehow put on the back burner. There's never a dull moment. While stressing over the cares of everyone else, then comes the extra stress of menopause. When it comes, it throws you completely off. For some women, this isn't good. Your emotions are on a roller coaster ride and you just want to get off. Some days you are up and some days you are down. Some days you don't know if you are coming or going. Some days, you want to pull your hair out and just scream.

> "The woman in your life may be experiencing some of this "craziness." It's a little scary because you don't know if you need to get professional help or if it will just pass."

There are days that you believe that you really are crazy and you are going to lose it. Some days you're screaming at your spouse and children, not knowing why you're screaming.

Menopause is overwhelming and frustrating. You can't understand what's going on within you and everything in you seems crazy. I believe that, for some women, a professional doctor or some type of professional help is essential. There has to be some type of balance, and the only way to find it is to involve a professional third party. A lot of people refuse to get help because they don't want to be labeled crazy, but it's crazy *not* to get the help that is needed. Sometimes third party insight is the best help you can get.

Mood swings are another part of the rollercoaster ride. According to WebMD, "Changes in estrogen levels and drops in progesterone levels may cause increased irritability and moodiness." There are times when I'm moody and irritable without me even knowing it. It takes my husband or children to bring it to my attention, and then I feel small, ashamed and embarrassed, because it's not who I am or a part of my make up.

One more thing I'd like to share with you is, loss of memory. This is a touchy subject for me because my father had Alzheimer's. So just the thought of me forgetting something or losing my memory is a big issue, and it becomes too much for me. I had another sigh of relief when I found out that memory loss was a symptom of menopause. Memory loss is a part of getting older, but for me, my thoughts were, "Not while I'm in my 40s!" My husband would ask me to do something and when he got home he'd ask if I did it, and my response would be, "I forgot." Now, after several times of saying those two words, he would get very angry with me, but I honestly would have forgotten. So we came up with the idea of me writing the things that he wanted me to do down. Well, that only worked when I would remember to write them down.

There are so many things and issues that come with this change of life. For some, there are no symptoms or changes, but for countless others, there's so much going on. I asked some women about menopause and they don't have a single problem, but for others, they're pulling their hair out. But with God's help, I believe any issue in life, including menopause, can be worked out for the good.

Focus on Love

When things get a little "crazy" and it seems like you can't take any more; read this scripture, which reminds us to always demonstrate the true character of love.

"⁴Love endures with patience and serenity, love is kind and thoughtful, and is not jealous or envious; love does not brag and is not proud or arrogant. ⁵It is not rude; it is not self-seeking, it is not provoked [nor overly sensitive and easily angered]; it does not take into account a wrong endured. ⁶It does not rejoice at injustice, but rejoices with the truth [when right and truth prevail]. ⁷Love bears all things [regardless of what comes], believes all things [looking for the best in each one], hopes all things [remaining steadfast during difficult times], endures all things [without weakening]. ⁸Love never fails [it never fades nor ends]..." 1 Corinthians 13:4-8 (Amplified Bible)

Chapter Five
WEIGHT ON!!

Menopause comes with a lot of changes and, at times, it seems so difficult and frustrating. Women generally put on a little weight as we began to age. You know the saying, "old age spread." During the process of menopause, I've experienced added weight to the weight I was already trying to get rid of. Unfortunately, weight-gain is an absolute in menopause. As WomentoWomen.com put it:

"Weight-gain becomes more complex during menopause; it's no longer simply, 'calories in, calories out.' As a woman transitions into perimenopause and menopause, her ovaries make fewer sex hormones, and this experience causes hormonal imbalance. Her body may respond by trying to protect itself. Its preferred method of protection is to store fat, especially around the waist, hips, and thighs. Fat stored in these areas also produces more estrogen, which in turn, leads to more fat production. The more estrogen deficient, the more it seems that the fat continues to accumulate around the hips and thighs. However, despite these changes taking place in her body, she can still achieve a healthy weight. Excellent nutrition and lower carbohydrates helps women balance their hormones and heal naturally."

One of the best things you can do to help is to encourage your girl to eat well! It's important she eats foods that will naturally speed up her metabolism. It's harder to get the weight off once everything slows down. I am currently trying to fight the bulge. I gave birth to five children; four of them are twins. I can no longer blame my weight gain on having two sets of twins, because the last set of twins are 13 now, but that was my excuse for years. Now that I am menopausal, it's been a struggle to get the weight off. That's when my husband and I decided to change the way we eat, not temporarily, but a lifestyle change, which means permanently.

> "...she needs to be encouraged like never before. This is the time to think of activities that you can do together that will benefit you both, such as walking, jogging, bike riding, and swimming. Whatever it takes to help make it through this challenging time."

The woman in your life may be frustrated with the extra weight and she needs to be encouraged like never before. This is the time to think of activities that you can do together that will benefit you both, such as walking, jogging, bike riding, and swimming. Whatever it takes to help make it through this challenging time.

A Prayer to Overcome the Effects of Menopause

(Pray this prayer. Insert your significant other's name in the blank.)

Father,

I declare that _____ will overcome ALL side effects of menopause, including fatigue and weight gain. Father, energize her body and give her the desire to make healthy meal choices when she is eating and shopping for food. Give her the wisdom she needs to plan and prepare healthy meals, and help her to enjoy them. Lord, let her know that you are right there with her every step of the way. Help me to not be critical of any shortcomings she may have. But give me the perfect words to encourage her and the strength to support her during this time. Give her the courage and strength to walk through this great journey and to be victorious. In the Mighty Name of Jesus…Amen!!

Chapter Six
HANG IN THERE!!

Again, the symptoms of menopause can cause challenges in your marriage and relationships. First and foremost, hang in there! Things may get worse before they get better. You must be equipped with some essential tools in order to make it through this process without losing your mind. In order to successfully make it through this trying time in your life, here are some sure tools that will help.

You will need:

1. Jesus   4. Patience   7. Prayer

2. Jesus   5. Patience   8. Prayer

3. Jesus   6. Patience   9. Prayer

10. More of Jesus, more patience, more prayer, and a WHOLE LOT OF UNDERSTANDING!!!

I know that menopause is a bit overwhelming for men as well. It's something that's happening to your woman, but it's overtaking you in the process. It's easy to want to give up and throw in the towel, especially when you don't have an understanding of what's going on. I have to say it again—**communication is key**. If you don't have a clue to what's going on, then you can't use your God-given gift to solve or fix problems. Menopause can cause you to feel helpless and so confused, but to overcome this phase with your significant other; knowledge is power.

It would be good to find some kind of outlet. Maybe try hanging out with some brothers or forming a support group with men who are going through the same thing. This could be a good way to vent to someone about the challenges you're facing. It's important to have a group of brothers to talk to and help you figure out ways to deal with the situation and better your relationship.

There are times when my husband is totally confused, and sometimes it leads to stress and misunderstandings because he doesn't understand what's happening or how to fix it. Menopause can stir up some things and cause disturbances in your relationship, but with knowledge and understanding, you'll be equipped to handle and go through any problem that comes with this GREAT "change" in you and your special lady's life.

A Prayer for Marriages

"Dear Lord, I pray for every couple that is going through menopause. I declare that they will experience peace, love, and understanding during this season in their in lives. I pray for increased strength, hope, and patience. When frustration sets in; I declare that joy and laughter will be their way of escape. I declare that the communication between the two of them will be increased above measure. I pray that they will intentionally invest daily in their relationship and grow in grace. In Jesus' name. Amen."

- Author Lelitia Lane

About the Author

Author Lelitia Lane is a native of Atlanta, Georgia. She graduated with honors from Beulah Heights University, where she received a Bachelor of Arts Degree in Biblical Education.

She is a licensed, ordained minister who loves to teach, preach and hear the Gospel of Jesus Christ. She is married to an awesome man of God, Pastor Roland Lane Jr. Lelitia and her husband serve alongside Pastor Gerald Jennings at *Love Outreach Worship Center* in Atlanta, Georgia.

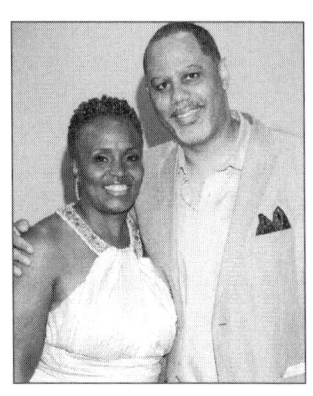

Author Lelitia Lane and her husband, Pastor Roland Lane Jr.

Lelitia is blessed with many gifts and talents. Singing has been her most dominant gift. Now, she has stepped up to embrace a gift that had been lying dormant for a while. Writing has become her new passion, and her first book, "Men-On-Pause," is evidence of that. She believes that writing her first book, and the many others that will follow, is a part of her purpose for this season in her life.

Lelitia is also passionate about working with youth. She is the founder and executive director of the *Good Girls Club*, a mentoring program for teenage girls (ages 11-15) who are "too old for toys, but too young for boys."

Among the greatest gifts she has been given are she and her husband's eight beautiful children, which out of the eight, they have two sets of twins!

To contact Lelitia for booking or inquiries, please send an email to **lelitia.lane@gmail.com**.

REFERENCES

Streicher, Lauren, MD. "The Cold Facts About Hot Flashes." The Dr. Oz Show. http://www.doctoroz.com/blog/lauren-streicher-md/cold-facts-about-hot-flashes/. (Retrieved November 2016).

Birch, Jenna. "10 Foods That Boost Your Libido (and 3 That Kill It)." Fitness Magazine. https://www.fitnessmagazine.com/mind-body/sex/libido-boosting-foods/. (Retrieved September 2016).

Healthy Women. "Intimacy Without Intercourse" Healthy Women. http://www.healthywomen.org/CONTENT/ARTICLE/INTIMACY-WITHOUT-INTERCOURSE?/. (Retrieved July 2016).

WebMD. "The Basics of Menopause." WebMD. https://www.webmd.com/menopause/guide/menopause-basics#1/. (Retrieved April 2016).

WebMD. "Menopause Overview & Facts" WebMD. https://www.webmd.com/menopause/guide/menopause-overview-facts/. (Retrieved October 2016).

Sharon, Stills, Dr (reviewed). "Top 10 menopause myths — busted!" Women's Health Network. https://www.womenshealthnetwork.com/menopause-and-perimenopause/menopause-myths.aspx/. (Retrieved March 2016).

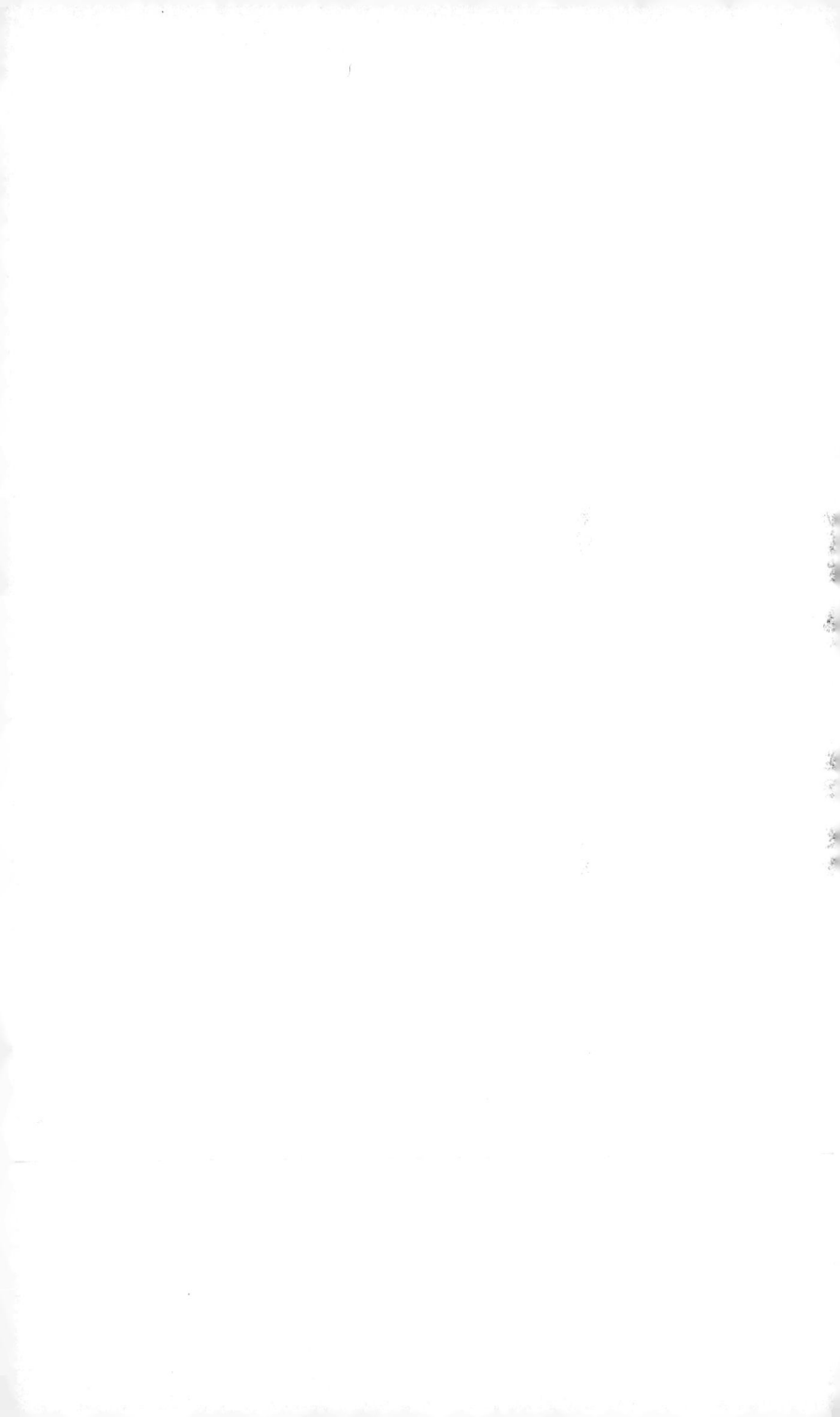

Printed in Great Britain
by Amazon